SHE SAID HE SAID

CONSENT WHILE DRINKING... FRAGMENTED MEMORIES

MARSHALL SMITH M.D.
FORENSIC PSYCHIATRIST

SHE SAID
HE SAID

CONSENT WHILE DRINKING...
FRAGMENTED MEMORIES

MARSHALL H. SMITH, M.D.
BOARD CERTIFIED FORENSIC PSYCHIATRIST

Copyright © 2019 Dr. Marshall Smith
She Said He Said
Consent While Drinking...
Fragmented Memories
By Dr. Marshall Smith

ISBN-13: 978-1091213104 (Paperback)

All rights reserved.

No part of this publication may be reproduced, distributed, or transmitted in any form or by any means, including photocopying, recording, or other electronic or mechanical methods, without the prior written permission of the publisher, except in the case of brief quotations embodied in critical reviews and certain other noncommercial uses permitted by copyright law.

Formerly titled *Sex While Intoxicated: Crime or Not* published in 2015.

Dr. Marshall Smith
alcoholexpert4u@yahoo.com

Manuscript Services by
Rogena Mitchell-Jones, Literary Editor
www.rogenamitchell.com

DISCLAIMER

The information provided in this book is designed to provide helpful information on the subjects discussed. This book is not meant to be used, nor should it be used, to diagnose or treat any medical condition. **This book is not intended as a substitute for the medical advice of an evaluating physician.**

The reader should regularly consult a physician in matters relating to his/her health and particularly with respect to any symptoms that may require diagnosis or medical attention.

Similarly, this book is not intended as a substitute for the legal advice of an attorney. It is not intended to support the prosecution or defense in actual cases, but is intended to provide general information to the general public. The author is not responsible for any specific health or legal needs that may require the assistance of a physician or attorney, and is not liable for any damages or negative consequences from any treatment, action, application or preparation, to any person reading or following the information in this book.

The purpose of the book is to increase awareness about the effects of alcohol on the human brain in effort to decrease the number of alcohol-related incidents.

Readers should be aware that the book is designed to provide general information and is not to be considered as consultative medical or legal services. It is sold with the understanding that the author's primary purpose is awareness and prevention. The author is not rendering any type of psychological, legal, or any other kind of professional consultation.

CONTENTS

1. Imagine This 1
2. Why I Decided to Write This Book 5
3. How Your Life May Change if Someone Rapes You When You are Too Intoxicated to Prevent it From Happening 11
4. How Your Life Will Change if You Are Accused and Convicted of Having Sex With Someone Who Says They Were Too Drunk to Consent 17
5. How Drinking Alcohol Leads to Intoxication and Why People Behave Certain Ways When They Drink 23
6. Why do Some People say They Cannot Remember Things They did After a Night of Drinking? 33
7. Why do Some People Fall Asleep or Pass Out After Drinking and Is It Okay to Have Sex With Someone Who Is Sleeping? 43
8. Can I Have Sex With Someone if We Both Have Been Drinking or Is It a Crime? 49
9. What Options Do I Have if, After a Night of Drinking, I Know I Have Been Raped? 57
10. What Should I Do If I Am Being Accused of Having Intercourse with Someone Who Says They Were Too Drunk to Consent? 62
11. Advice From The Author 67
12. Dr. Marshall Smith 73

1

IMAGINE THIS

Imagine you have been selected to be on the jury for a trial. For some of you, this might be a scary idea. You may have watched shows on television where a trial was being shown and even thought it might be cool to actually be a member of the jury. You may have even wondered how the jury came up with a particular verdict because, as you watched the trial, you may have seen things differently and came up with the opposite verdict. So now, here's your opportunity in real life to be on an actual jury that's going to decide the fate of the person who is on trial.

You may have found it difficult to sleep the night before trial because you were nervous and anticipating how it was going to feel as you walked into the courtroom the next morning. You wake up that morning and wonder why you are making frequent trips to the bathroom.

As you walk into the courtroom, you see the judge sitting there wearing a black robe, you see lawyers who will defend the person on trial, and lawyers who will try to convince you the person on trial is guilty.

You also see people sitting in the back of the courtroom, and you wonder who they are. Are they friends or family members of the people involved in the case, or are they just people who didn't have anything else to do that day, so they decided to come watch a trial? Whoever they are, it seems all of them are looking directly at you as you take your seat in the jury section. You have seen this scenario so many times on television, but for some reason, it all seems so different in real life. Everyone in the courtroom knows you will be one of the people who will decide if the person on trial is guilty or not guilty.

The case involves someone who says they were drunk and unable to give consent to have sex when the person on trial took advantage of them and raped them. The person on trial said the sex was consensual. How could their stories be completely opposite? Someone must be lying. You ask yourself how you will be able to tell who's telling the truth, because you have no special training in that area, and you are not a human lie detector.

As the trial begins, the judge asks the lawyers if they want to make any opening statements, and both sets of lawyers try to convince you that their client is telling the truth and the other person is lying. Both sets of lawyers sound so convincing, and at that point, you have no idea who to believe. The trial starts and you listen to the witnesses and consider all the evidence presented. At the conclusion of the trial, the judge gives you some instructions to consider as you leave the courtroom to discuss the case with the other jury members.

Hopefully, based on all the evidence, you are convinced one way or the other, and your decision is easy.

What if you are not convinced and you are unsure if the person on trial is guilty or not guilty? Well, the judge said you had to be convinced beyond a reasonable doubt that the person on trial is guilty; otherwise, you had to find them not guilty. You think you understand what beyond a reasonable doubt means, but you have never been asked to decide something beyond a reasonable doubt before. How do you know what's reasonable and what's unreasonable?

Do all the jury members have the same understanding of what's reasonable and what's beyond reasonable? The pressure continues to build inside of you because you don't want to mess this up and make the wrong decision.

Do you tell the other jury members that you really don't understand what beyond a reasonable doubt means? What will they think of you if you say you are undecided and unsure of what beyond a reasonable doubt really means?

Should you just guess because it's been a long trial and everyone else has already made his or her decision? Would you be able to live with yourself if you make the wrong decision and let a rapist go free, or even worse, find an innocent person guilty and send them to prison?

Now imagine you are the person who says they were too drunk to consent to sex and got raped, or imagine you are the person accused of rape and on trial. What would you want from the jury? Would you want someone like you to be on the jury? How would you feel if the jury gets it all wrong and finds the person who raped you not guilty or wrongfully convicts you of rape when you know the sex was consensual?

I hope you saw yourself sitting in that courtroom as you read. Did your imagination take you there? As you read further, I hope you gain a better understanding of the effects of alcohol on the brain so if you ever find yourself in a courtroom for a case involving an alcohol-related sexual assault, you will be there to support a friend or loved one and not as the alleged victim or the accused.

2

WHY I DECIDED TO WRITE THIS BOOK

Over the past twenty years, I have come in contact with many individuals who abused alcohol and either became victims of alcohol-related non-consensual sex or were accused of having sex with someone who was too intoxicated to give consent. To be clear up front, I am not referring to people who prey upon others intentionally for their own gratification. I think people who prey on others should be prosecuted to the fullest extent of the law and punished accordingly if found guilty of the charges.

Determining how many alcohol-related sexual assaults occur from year to year is almost impossible. Many people choose not to report an assault, and others are confused about whether or not they were assaulted and decide to keep it to themselves. Some say each year over 60,000 students between the ages of 18 and 24 are victims of alcohol-related sexual assault, and up to fifteen percent of those are under the legal drinking age. Others say more than fifty percent of college-age sexual assaults are associated with alcohol use. If we include others outside of that age group and include the general population, the number of alcohol-related sexual assaults increases significantly.

I believe you will agree with me that determining the actual number of sexual assaults should not be our focus, but preventing each and every assault should be our priority. One assault is too many, and I believe through education and awareness, we can empower potential victims of improper alcohol-related behavior to avoid the negative and life-changing consequences.

I have spoken many times in various settings on the effects of alcohol on the brain, and people often tell me they learned a great deal from hearing me speak. Many have said to me that after hearing me talk about the harmful effects of alcohol, they were going to change their drinking patterns before something bad happened to them. They felt lucky something had not already happened to ruin their lives.

As a forensic psychiatrist, I am often called as an expert witness in court cases involving alcohol and the ability or lack of ability to consent to sex. In those settings, I am asked to explain to the jury how alcohol affects the brain, and potentially clear up misconceptions related to a person's ability to function while under the influence of alcohol.

Although most people have a general knowledge about alcohol intoxication, they are unaware of how alcohol can impair a person's memory and how alcohol is associated with an individual's ability to consent to have sex. I have seen so many lives wrecked where alcohol was involved. I've spoken to many alcohol-related rape victims who have difficulty going on with their lives because, after being raped, they have problems with anxiety and depression. Some of them have even attempted suicide because they were unable to deal with the trauma associated with being raped.

Contrarily, I have also spoken to many people who were accused of having sex with someone who said they were too drunk to consent. Some were found guilty and sent to prison while others went to court and were found not guilty. Unfortunately, alcohol-related sexual assault court cases are far too common. In a lot of cases, because there are no witnesses to what actually happened on the day or night in question, the jury decision can have one of several results. These results range from a true rapist found guilty, an innocent person mistakenly found guilty, an innocent person rightfully found not guilty, or a guilty person found not guilty and cleared to return home and to potentially rape someone else.

In the majority of court cases where I have been involved, I respect the jury's decision and do not envy them and the difficult job they have. They will decide the fate of the accused, and based on the details of the case, they may have a difficult time agreeing on a verdict. Going to court is often difficult for the alleged victim and the accused. I hope by reading this book, you will get a better understanding of what it may be like for a rape victim to take the witness stand in a courtroom to explain what happened to them. I also hope you can get a glimpse of what it may be like to be the accused.

The best scenario is to avoid finding yourself in court as either the alleged victim or the accused. How can this be achieved? I wrote this book to educate the general public on the devastating effects alcohol can have on a person's ability to make decisions and ultimately consent to having sex. My goal in writing this book is to prevent someone from becoming a victim of an alcohol-related sexual assault and to prevent other well-intentioned people from carelessly getting in a position where they are accused of alcohol-related sexual assault.

Being raped or falsely accused of rape are always life changing and devastating to all involved. Not only do these situations affect the victim and the accused, but their families, friends, and loved ones are also affected. Often times, the people involved are young adults who did well in high school, are hard-working, law-abiding citizens, have aspirations to further their education, and are generally good people. They come from loving and nurturing families, have the potential to become anything they want to in life, and would not intentionally put themselves in a compromising situation.

That is why the information in this book is so valuable. I purposefully limited the information contained in this book to the basic facts and topics I felt would be most helpful to you. As you will see, this is not a novel consisting of hundreds of pages to entertain you, nor does it contain a considerable amount of scientific or technical terms that can be confusing and hard to understand. The book was written as a handbook or teaching tool with the sole purpose of preventing alcohol-related sexual assaults.

My intention is to get straight to the point so you can read this book in one or two sittings, to increase your awareness about the effects of alcohol on the brain, and how alcohol can interrupt you having a good time and turn the perfect evening into your worst nightmare. I have used several scenarios in an attempt to make the information more realistic, and I'm sure you will relate to some of the details mentioned in the scenarios.

I wrote this book to help all groups of people. If you

are a teenager still in high school, this book is for you. If you are a college student, this book is for you. If you are a young adult in the workplace or military, this book is for you. If you are a brother, sister, mother, father, child, friend, mentor, grandparent, or someone who just cares about someone else, this book is for you. You see my point? This book is for everyone.

I hope this book enlightens you about the effects of alcohol on human beings so you don't let alcohol ruin your dreams. I want you to understand the negative consequences associated with being sexually assaulted, so if you drink, you will drink responsibly. I also want you to know how alcohol can affect your judgment and cause you to make poor decisions that may lead to you finding yourself standing in a courtroom while the jury convicts you and sends you to prison for many years. If you are a family member or friend, show your love and empower your loved ones with the information in this book.

If you are a parent, I beg you to share this book with your children. Use it as a way to educate them on the debilitating effects of alcohol. Wouldn't you rather sit with your loved one, proactively preparing them as you have done their entire life? The alternative would be sitting with them in a hospital emergency room while they are being examined after an assault or sitting with them in a prison visitation room after they have been convicted of having sex with someone who they thought had the ability to consent. You have spent a lot of time and energy rearing your children, and I know you want the best for them. Empower them with the information in this book so they can take care of themselves and continue to have a happy and successful life.

Too many people live the rest of their lives suffering from the adverse consequences of poor decisions made while under the influence of alcohol. The information in this book is for everyone. Regardless of your age or position in life, I hope you find something in this book to either help yourself or help someone you love or care for. Together, I'm confident we can make a difference. I hope you enjoy reading the book, and I wish you much success and happiness.

3

HOW YOUR LIFE MAY CHANGE IF SOMEONE RAPES YOU WHEN YOU ARE TOO INTOXICATED TO PREVENT IT FROM HAPPENING

SCENARIO # 1

A very responsible and well-respected young lady decides to go to a local restaurant within walking distance of her home with a few friends of both genders to celebrate her twenty-first birthday. After a few drinks and dinner, they decide to walk down the street to one of their favorite bars. Because she is now twenty-one, she drinks more alcohol than she intended to drink. Although she had a good time, before leaving to return home, she is unable to walk without assistance and the room seems to be spinning.

One of her friends essentially has to carry her home because she is unable to walk. Once inside her apartment, she gets into bed and is barely awake. Her friend wants to have sex with her and she tells him no. He persists and she continues to tell him no.

Because of her level of intoxication, she is physically unable to fight him off, and he undresses her from the *waist down and has intercourse with her against her will. She cries the entire time because she cannot believe this is happening to her. She reports the incident the next day, and eight months later, after a lengthy investigation, he is convicted of rape and sent to prison.*

Being raped is probably one of the most devastating things one can go through in life. The young lady in the scenario was celebrating her birthday and then realized she had too much to drink. She knew she needed help getting home and decided to ask a friend she trusted for assistance. She felt safe with him and probably never imagined he would take advantage of her. I want to make a huge point here, so please read carefully, and appreciate the importance of age. Notice she was twenty-one-years-old, which means she was of legal age to drink.

In many of the cases I'm involved with in court, the alleged victim and the accused are under twenty-one-years-old and should not have been drinking in the first place. Depending on where you live, the legal drinking age may be different. I wish I could only say don't drink until you are of the legal age, but we must keep it real. Some of you reading this book are probably underage, and I'm sure some of you drink. You probably know other underage drinkers, and some of you probably have no intentions of waiting until you reach the legal age.

It's kind of like telling someone who is sexually active to not have sex until they are married. Abstinence may be the safest and recommended course of action, but let's not fool ourselves into thinking that most sexually active people are going to stop having sex just because someone tells them they should wait until they are married.

Well, the same rationale goes for underage drinkers. Underage drinkers know they are underage, and they also know there will be negative consequences if they get caught. Most, however, continue to drink because they know other underage drinkers, and no one believes they will get caught. So, for the record, if you are underage and you drink, I want you to stop today. I can hear some of you saying, "Yeah, right, Dr. Smith. I like to drink, and I'm not waiting until I'm twenty-one." Perhaps, after you read the book, you may think twice about underage drinking, or at least have a better appreciation of how alcohol can damage your brain.

Regardless of your age, if you become a victim of an alcohol-related sexual assault, your life will never be the same. The victim in the scenario is a female, and the rapist is a male. Some of you may be surprised to hear this, but males get raped, too. When people hear about someone getting raped, most assume the victim is a female and the rapist is a male. Some of my cases involve male victims and the perpetrators have been other males as well as females.

The main point to understand here is a person of either gender can be a victim of rape just as a person of either sex can be a rapist. Being raped can have lasting physical and psychological effects.

Although sometimes there are no visible signs of rape, some of the potential physical manifestations can include: contracting sexually transmitted diseases like gonorrhea, herpes, chlamydia, syphilis, or HIV; getting tears inside and outside of the vaginal area; getting tears inside and outside of the anal area; unwanted pregnancy; bruises on the head, face, neck, arms, abdomen, genital region, legs, and back.

I have treated several patients who actually got pregnant after being raped. They all struggled with what they should do about the pregnancy. Some knew from the beginning they were going to get an abortion and kept the pregnancy a secret from their family and friends.

Others didn't believe in abortion but did not want to have a child that would remind them of the rape. Some of my patients, who actually decided to have an abortion, felt a tremendous amount of guilt, and never forgave themselves for having the abortion.

Can you imagine the dilemma they were in? One of my patients is still suffering from the trauma associated with the rape, and it has been over twenty years since it actually happened. She went to a party when she was 18 years old, had one drink, and woke up to someone raping her. Even though it has been over twenty years, she still breaks down and cries every time she talks about it.

With the exception of a few of the physical manifestations mentioned above, most physical manifestations resolve with time and appropriate treatment. Unfortunately, the potential psychological manifestations can be just as hard or even harder to live with.

Unlike physical signs of trauma, psychological signs are often invisible to others. I use the word trauma because rape is a traumatic experience that can affect your mental health for the rest of your life. The quality of life for most rape victims is significantly reduced, which causes them to seek assistance from a mental health professional.

As a psychiatrist, I have evaluated and treated many patients, both female and male, who were victims of sexual assault. Most of those patients experienced significant anxiety and depression that interfered with the quality of their interpersonal relationships with family members, friends, and coworkers.

Many of them were diagnosed with Posttraumatic Stress Disorder, PTSD. PTSD is a trauma-related disorder that can develop after experiencing a traumatic event like being raped. Some of the symptoms can include nightmares about the assault that significantly interfere with sleep and make people afraid to go to sleep, avoidance of people and places that may remind them of the attack, or feelings that they cannot trust anyone. The patient can feel they are a bad person and blame themselves. They may be unable to feel love or experience happiness. Additionally, they may experience chest discomfort, numbness, tingling sensations in their hands, shortness of breath, dizziness, nausea, choking sensations, sweating, and trembling. Some may feel as if they are losing their mind, be on edge all the time, or even yell at loved ones about little things.

Can you imagine how life would be for you if you experienced some of those symptoms every day? Many patients with PTSD are unable to function in school or on the job, and they don't even feel comfortable in their own homes.

They may have difficulty with intimate relationships because they don't feel comfortable hugging, kissing, or having sexual intercourse with their significant other.

Just think about it.

What do you think would happen if you were in a relationship where every time your significant other touches you, it takes you back to the time you were raped and you withdraw from any form of affection and intimacy?

How do you think your significant other would understand and tolerate a relationship that lacks intimacy? The relationship may be unfulfilling and miserable for both of you because you cannot adjust to the pain associated with intimacy and so you avoid it at all cost.

As a result, it is not uncommon for victims of rape to experience unhealthy interpersonal relationships and failed marriages. Some people with PTSD begin to abuse illicit drugs and to engage in self-destructive behavior. Because of the pain and impact those symptoms have on their quality of life, some people with PTSD think about committing suicide, make suicide attempts, and unfortunately, some have actually ended their lives by successfully committing suicide.

Treatment for PTSD is very effective, and usually consists of either talk therapy alone or talk therapy in combination with medication therapy. If you think you may have PTSD or if you know someone you think may have PTSD, help is available. You don't have to suffer through the symptoms by yourself. Many of my patients said their reluctance to seek treatment initially was because they didn't think anyone would understand, and they felt like no one else was experiencing anything similar. After engaging in treatment, most regain their sense of control and go on to live productive and happy lives.

4

HOW YOUR LIFE WILL CHANGE IF YOU ARE ACCUSED AND CONVICTED OF HAVING SEX WITH SOMEONE WHO SAYS THEY WERE TOO DRUNK TO CONSENT

SCENARIO # 2

A twenty-two-year-old college senior attends a fraternity party on campus. He just completed final exams and is anticipating graduation in a couple of weeks. He also recently found out that he was going to be hired into his dream job after graduation and wants to celebrate. He sees a female friend at the party. He has known her for about three years. They have been interested in each other and have actually talked about dating in the past. On that night, they have a few drinks and enjoy each other's company at the party. They both get a little tipsy, and she kisses him and asks him if he wants to go back to his apartment. They leave the party arm in arm and walk to his apartment. They enter his room, and after briefly talking, they continue making out.

Everything seems fine to him, and it appears they both are into each other. They both take off their own clothes and engage in what he considers consensual *sex. After they finish, she tells him goodbye, gets dressed, and leaves his apartment. As she is leaving, one of her boyfriend's best friend's sees her exit the apartment, and confronts her. She feels embarrassed for cheating on her boyfriend and is worried he will find out.*

Feeling she was taken advantage of because she was intoxicated, she reports the incident to the campus police. She says she thinks she was raped because she had been drinking and was too drunk to consent. The senior gets arrested and is charged with having sex with her when she was unable to consent due to the effects of the alcohol.

Believe it or not, this scenario is real life for a lot of people. Some of you may think he deserves to be charged with sexual assault because you believe that after one drink a person is not able to consent. We will explore that concept later, but first, we must explore how that allegation will affect that senior's life. According to him, they were having a good time and enjoying each other's company. He admitted he was attracted to her, and she also admitted she was attracted to him. They had even thought about dating. When they left the party to return to his apartment, he did not feel he was taking advantage of her.

During the entire evening, he was very respectful towards her and thought he was a gentleman. He enjoyed making out with her and thought she was totally consenting. Prior to her leaving his apartment after having sex, he gave her a kiss and told her how much he enjoyed spending the night with her. She said she also had a good time and told him she would see him later.

So what happened? Why did she report him to the

campus police a few days later? Was she too intoxicated to consent, or did she need an excuse for cheating on her boyfriend? Should he have known not to have sex with her? Well, whatever the truth is, his life will never be the same. What do you think will happen after graduation?

Do you think he will be able to graduate with legal charges pending? Probably not. What about that super job offer he was looking forward to starting? What will his employer think when they find out he is facing rape charges? Will they hold the job for him or fire him before he even gets started? What would you do if you were the employer? The notification might go something like this: "Hello, Mr. or Mrs. CEO of the company, my graduation has been put on hold because I'm facing rape charges. I know this sounds bad, but I'm innocent. I have an attorney, and he said the investigation and trial will probably take anywhere from six months to a year.

"I'm sure I will be found not guilty, so will you hold my job for a year until this whole ordeal is over? I hope I will graduate a year from now and be found not guilty of the charges, but my lawyer said there was a possibility I will be convicted of the charges, not graduate, be registered as a sex offender, and go to prison for a long time. I hope it doesn't happen because I didn't do anything wrong. Thank you for understanding, and please hold my job for me until all of this is cleared up."

Ok, now what would you do if you were the employer?

Graduating from college and getting that job is the least of his worries at this point. Depending on the state you live in, most rape convictions carry a sentence of three to ten years in a state prison and registration as a sex offender for the rest of your life.

Now let's go back to the day of the arrest, and let me walk you through what your life may consist of if you are alleged to have had sex with someone when that person was too intoxicated to give consent.

First of all, you will probably be arrested and brought to the police station. The arrest will likely involve you being placed in handcuffs and directed to a police car. Your family and or friends will probably watch as you walk with your hands handcuffed behind your back. That experience will likely be extremely embarrassing to you. Next, at the police station, you will be asked to speak to the detectives so they can hear your side. You may have an attorney already, but if you don't, they will tell you that you have a right to a lawyer. That process usually takes several hours, and depending on the situation, you may be allowed to leave after that or you may have to go to jail until you can see a judge.

At some point, you will be told that you are being formally charged with rape, and you may even have to pay a fee to be released from jail. The amount of that fee could range from $10,000 to $20,000, or even more. Some of you may not have difficulty finding $10,000, but many of you probably have no idea of how to come up with that amount of money. You probably don't have it, and your family may not have it either.

Now that you are out of jail, what will you do while the investigation is ongoing? How are you going to pay for your attorney? Some attorney's charge more than others do, but it would not be unusual to pay an attorney over $25,000 to take your case. We have not even talked about the emotional pain and suffering you will be subjected to throughout this process, but financially, it would not be unrealistic for you to spend well over $30,000 to defend yourself.

After the investigation, you find yourself sitting in court on trial for rape. People in the courtroom are looking at you as if you are already guilty, and you are scared because you know if the jury finds you guilty, you will go to prison. You sit there in the courtroom as the prosecutor tells the jury how bad a person you are because you raped someone who did not have the ability to consent. Your fate is in the hands of the jury, and you can do nothing about it.

Your 'friend' takes the witness stand and tells her side of the story. You sit there in disbelief as she describes the events that took place in your apartment on the night in question. You don't remember things happening the way she is describing them, and you know you would never have taken advantage of her. She says she was intoxicated to the point of not being able to consent to sex and that you took advantage of her. Her recollection of the events that happened that night is entirely different from what you remember.

At the end of the trial, you stand up as the judge asks the jury if they have reached a verdict. Your heart is pounding and sweat is forming on your forehead as you listen to the jury foreman announce the verdict. Your entire life now depends on one or two words—GUILTY or NOT GUILTY. As you stand there in anticipation, those who care about you and love you are also nervous and scared. Their hearts are pounding just as much as yours because they know if you are found guilty, you will go to prison, and your hopes and dreams will probably never become a reality.

As you stand there hoping to hear the words NOT

GUILTY, suddenly you hear the jury foreman say your name and inform you the court has found you GUILTY. You hear your family members standing behind you start to cry, and you almost collapse because you cannot believe you are now a convicted rapist on your way to prison. You begin to ask yourself how can this be. Are you dreaming or is this reality? Your loved ones are sobbing now because they know you are a good person and that you would never rape someone. They know you don't deserve to go to prison, but there is nothing they can do to help you now.

You start to cry as you are put into handcuffs and led out of the courtroom. In a matter of seconds, you went from being accused and thinking there was no way you would be convicted to now being a convicted rapist and sex offender. As you sit alone in your small jail cell that night, dressed in your orange jumpsuit, you are still in disbelief. You find out you are sentenced to eight years, and within a few days, you are transported from the jail to state prison.

Use your imagination as you consider what you will encounter over the next eight years of your life.

Some of you may be saying this is not fair, but fair or not, this is a reality for some. I encourage you to continue reading this book so you can enhance your knowledge about the intoxicating effects of alcohol and ultimately avoid becoming a victim of an alcohol-related incident.

5

HOW DRINKING ALCOHOL LEADS TO INTOXICATION AND WHY PEOPLE BEHAVE CERTAIN WAYS WHEN THEY DRINK

Understanding how alcohol affects the human brain and human behavior is crucial. Many people drink alcoholic beverages without having an appreciation of how the alcohol may impact their ability to make good decisions. Every day, people find themselves in trouble with the police because of things they did while they were under the influence of alcohol. Perhaps one of the most common things people do after drinking is drive their vehicles. They don't realize how impaired they may be after just a few drinks, so they get behind the wheel and attempt to drive to their destinations.

I'm sure some of you who are reading this right now have driven after you have been drinking or know someone who drove their vehicle after drinking. We will talk about how alcohol leads to intoxication, and why people are unable to perform certain tasks after drinking, but first, I want to spend a few minutes on what may happen to you if you drink and drive. Close to one million people across the United States are arrested for driving while intoxicated (DUI) each year, and close to 10,000 people die each year secondary to alcohol-related traffic accidents.

This may surprise you, but people under twenty-one years of age make up a significant number of those arrests and deaths. If you are arrested for drinking and driving, you will go to jail for up to a week, you will have to pay a fine that can be up to $500, your driver's license will be suspended for up to six months, and you may have to pay legal fees and court costs. Is it really worth it? Driving after having a few drinks may cost you your life, someone else's life, or land you in jail with fines and a criminal record that may prevent you from many opportunities in life.

Now I want to discuss why alcohol makes people feel intoxicated. This is not intended to be a scientific description involving the complex process of alcohol metabolism, and my intent is not to impress you with a lot of medical terminologies. That information is beyond the scope of this book but is available in textbooks and other resources if you are interested in a more in-depth explanation and understanding. People often say they want to get tipsy, wasted, smashed, tore-up, hammered, shit-faced, drunk, buzzed, sauced, fucked-up, and many other slangs, but basically, what they are describing is the way they want to feel when they drink enough alcohol.

There are many forms of alcoholic beverages, and most people are familiar with a variety of beers, wines, whiskeys, vodkas, gins, rums, tequilas, cognacs, scotches, and several others. Common drinks include beer alone, beer mixed with other things, rum and coke, vodka and tonic, whiskey and coke, various shots, gin and juice, and many others. The alcohol content in the different forms of drinks will differ, and some drinks have more alcohol in them than others. Some people enjoy the way the alcohol tastes and don't necessarily try to get intoxicated, but others know from the beginning they want to get a buzz and are going to drink until they feel buzzed.

Most don't understand in order to feel that way they will probably have to drink more alcohol than one body can efficiently process. The body has ways to deal with the alcohol as it moves from your mouth, down your esophagus, into your stomach, and then into your intestines. Most of the alcohol is absorbed into your body after it reaches your stomach and small intestines. Your liver is the primary organ that breaks down the alcohol so it does not become harmful to you. If you drink more alcohol than your liver can handle, the alcohol will build up in your bloodstream and travel to your brain.

Alcohol basically prevents or inhibits your brain from working properly, and has a depressing or dampening effect on your brain. In medical terminology, alcohol is a central nervous system depressant, and your central nervous system consists of your brain and your spinal cord. It doesn't take much alcohol for you to become impaired, and most people start feeling the effects of alcohol after having just one or two drinks. The first time you drink alcohol, you may become impaired after just having a few sips. More experienced drinkers can usually tolerate more drinks before they begin to feel intoxicated. A general and widely accepted concept is that your body can handle approximately one 12-ounce beer or one mixed drink per hour.

There is something known as binge drinking. Binge drinking is when someone drinks excessively over a short period of time. A commonly accepted definition of binge drinking is drinking five drinks for men and four drinks for women over two hours. People who binge drink can become intoxicated rapidly. There are other variables that must be considered and will influence your level of intoxication. If you are lighter weight, if you drink on an empty stomach, if you are a female, and if you are a relatively new drinker, you will probably become more intoxicated if you drink the same amount of alcohol as someone who weighs more than you, someone who drinks after eating a full meal, a male if you are a female, a more experienced drinker, and other factors based on your family's genes. I'm sure most of you have seen someone you thought was intoxicated. You may not have seen them drinking, but because of their behavior, you knew something wasn't right.

In many of the cases I have been involved with, people commonly think there are two ways to describe someone who has been drinking. They think a person is either drunk or not drunk. I've heard people say things like, "He was drunk and so he could not have known what he was doing," and "She was obviously drunk so she did not have the ability to consent." Well, it's not as simple as that, and rather than saying someone was drunk, determining his or her level of intoxication based on observed behavior is critical.

So what behaviors are associated with drinking alcohol and becoming intoxicated with alcohol?

Let's begin by describing the behavior of someone who is completely sober. Someone sober is probably going to be in control of his or her actions and based on their personality, they may be outgoing and assertive or shy and reserved. They will likely be able to participate in conversations and utilize good judgment in making decisions. These are the friends usually identified to be the designated driver because either they don't drink or they will not drink on a particular evening. Have you ever gone to a party with friends and decided to identify a designated driver even before the party begins? Why do people even think about having a designated driver in the first place?

The main reason is they know they are going to drink, and they also know more than likely, they will not be in any condition to drive. If you are planning to drink, take the time beforehand and make arrangements to have a designated driver. The designated driver will protect you from making poor decisions that may lead to you getting behind the wheel when you are impaired and unable to safely drive yourself home.

Now let's talk about those of you who are going to be drinking. Here's a possible scenario: You get to the party and the music is sounding good. The lights are low and you are ready to party. You see your friends and everyone else is drinking. You get a drink and actually start to enjoy yourself. You are not intoxicated, and no one can tell that you even had a drink. You decide to get another drink, and now you are really relaxed and feeling good. At that moment, you are probably in a euphoric state, which basically means the alcohol is beginning to take effect on you. You are in total control of the situation and you are enjoying the company of your friends.

Well, it's been a few minutes, and now you decide to have another drink. So, for the sake of argument, let's say it's been about an hour now and you have your third drink. At this point, you may start doing and saying things that you normally would not do or say. Examples could include things like flirting with someone or telling things you wouldn't tell anyone when you are sober. Some people describe having 'liquid courage' at this level of intoxication because they may now have the courage to ask someone to dance when before they did not have the nerve. Some people may become very flirtatious or get kind of loud or obnoxious. You may want to take selfies to send to your friends, or you may want to text them to tell them how much you love and miss them.

Some of you may want to call them because you just know they would love to hear your voice. Oh, yeah. You are feeling good now. Guess what happens next? You are correct—it's time for drink number four. So it's been less than two hours since you arrived at the party and now you have had four drinks. If you are a female, you have officially met the criteria for binge drinking and may have started something that may lead you down a path you didn't intend to go down when you decided to go to the party. I know I said earlier that binge drinking for males was five drinks over two hours, so let's kick it up a notch.

If you are a male—you know, the macho man male who is there to party and show everyone how cool he is, you don't want to waste too much time, and now you have consumed five or six drinks in less than two hours. You may even be proud of the fact that you can drink more than your friends can, and may even challenge them to some of the more popular drinking games. You may even be trying to impress someone at the party, so you decide to show them how much of a man you are by drinking everyone else under the table.

Congratulations. You have also officially met the definition of binge drinking. So what behaviors might we see as we progress from the euphoric liquid courage stage? The excitement continues, and now you begin to notice your balance is a little off, you become less coordinated, and your judgment may be impaired. Your friends can definitely tell you are intoxicated now because, although you are still able to participate in conversations with them, some of your speech may be slurred. Your visual acuity may also be affected. The person you thought was extremely ugly and repulsive earlier in the evening has now suddenly become the most attractive and desirable person you have seen in your life.

You just have to have that person, and your friends are shocked to see you making out with your newfound soul mate. You may even be a little nauseated and feel like you have to vomit.

Some people continue to drink at this point because, even though they know they are intoxicated, their critical judgment is impaired, and for some reason, they feel like another drink is required. They order another drink, even after their friends tell them they have had enough, and they dismiss their friends' advice. They quickly finish the entire drink, and then shortly afterward, notice the room seems to be spinning.

They become a little confused and disoriented, their balance is really off now, and their gait is significantly impaired. Now their friends are really annoyed with them because they just vomited all over the table, or even worse, they actually vomited in someone's lap.

As their level of intoxication continues to increase, they may become stuporous and be unable to stand or walk. They may lose control of most bodily functions and become incontinent of urine and feces. Their respiratory drive and ability to breathe on their own may be compromised. They may even progress to being in a coma and eventually, can rapidly progress to respiratory arrest and death. Obviously, the progression of impairment is directly proportional to the amount of alcohol consumed and the amount of alcohol that gets into the bloodstream.

The amount of alcohol that enters the bloodstream can be calculated by doing a blood test, but how many people are going to stop partying and ask someone to draw blood to determine his or her level of intoxication? Certain behaviors are associated with specific blood alcohol concentrations, but realistically, you will not know what someone's blood alcohol concentration is unless they are evaluated in an emergency room.

To protect yourself and your friends, be familiar with the behavioral signs mentioned above, and intervene quickly if you see one of your friends becoming increasingly intoxicated. Know that at a certain point, their judgment will become impaired, and they may make poor choices that have negative consequences. If you recognize yourself getting intoxicated to a level where you are uncomfortable, stop drinking, and ask someone you can trust to help you get home. It would be best if you leave with a group of people to avoid being with an individual who may not have your best interest at heart. If you notice one of your friends seems more intoxicated than they should be, take the appropriate action to prevent them from making poor decisions. Do not let them drive and do not let them leave the party with someone who may take advantage of them.

This may sound like common sense and something that is easy to do, but often times, when people become intoxicated to the point where they are making poor choices they are unwilling to listen to those who care about them. They may have a false sense of being able to care for themselves and may think you are trying to control them. They may become upset with you, and even become combative or belligerent. The worst mistake you can make at that time is to get upset and allow your friend to have their way. It's easy to say something like this, "OK, I've been trying to help you because you are so drunk you cannot even stand up by yourself. Look at you slurring your speech and you even threw up all over the floor, but if you are going to be an ass about it and get mad at me for trying to help you, just go ahead and see what happens."

Some of you might be able to see yourself saying something like that to a friend after repeatedly getting cussed out and told to leave them alone. Just remember—they are intoxicated and probably don't even realize what they are saying. Don't take it personal, and try to attempt to take control of the situation. The best thing you can do is to remain with your friend and not leave them alone. If other friends are around, ask them to assist.

It's easier to take control of the situation if you have the assistance of a few friends. Your intoxicated friend might not realize they are about to make poor decisions that could result in their death.

If you see a friend who is so intoxicated they have passed out and are asleep, they may be unable to wake up and might have what's known as alcohol poisoning. Alcohol poisoning is a medical emergency, and your friend might stop breathing and die if medical help is not initiated.

In some instances, calling 911 may be required if you are unable to wake your friend up and it appears their breathing is very shallow and weak. You might be the friend who saves a life, prevents an intoxicated friend from getting raped, and prevents an intoxicated friend from being accused of having sex with someone who says he or she was too intoxicated to consent to sex. Over the years, I have spoken to many people who said they stood by and watched one of their friends become extremely drunk to the point where they thought their friend was going to die.

If you ever find yourself in this situation, have the courage to seek help, even to the point of calling 911 if you have to. Don't fail to act and then have to live with the guilt of knowing you actually had the opportunity to help prevent a friend from getting seriously hurt or losing their life. When in doubt, take the cautious approach and do the right thing. Be the friend who cares and who is not afraid to take action to avoid an adverse outcome.

6

WHY DO SOME PEOPLE SAY THEY CANNOT REMEMBER THINGS THEY DID AFTER A NIGHT OF DRINKING?

SCENARIO # 3

A nineteen-year-old boy goes to a party and challenges one of his friends to a beer pong competition. He consumes a total of ten beers over a two-hour period. He is excited to win the game and takes his shirt off to pound his chest. He then stands on the table and begins to dance. Everyone is clapping for him, and he decides to strip down to his underwear. He then jumps off the table into the crowd. After the party ends, against the advice of his friends, he drives home. He wakes up the next morning and remembers being at the party. He remembers playing beer pong and remembers dancing. He remembers taking his shirt off but has no recollection of taking his pants off or jumping off the table. He also has no memory of how he got home from the party. He sees his car in his garage and wonders how it got there.

I hope you realize his drinking meets the definition of binge drinking. Just for review purposes, remember that binge drinking is associated with many unwanted behaviors and negative aspects of drinking. For men, five or more drinks in a two-hour period and for women, four or more drinks in a two-hour period is considered binge drinking. If you binge drink, you are putting yourself at increased risk for an alcohol-related incident. Your blood alcohol concentration will elevate rapidly because your liver will not be able to adequately process and eliminate the increased amount of alcohol you consumed. Additionally, remember that the legal drinking age is twenty-one.

When people binge drink, they may quickly progress through the stages of intoxication and experience some or all of the behaviors associated with increasing levels of intoxication. Let's do a quick review of the different behaviors associated with increasing levels of alcohol consumption. No signs of drinking after having a few sips to one drink. Then, the relaxation and feeling good occurs. Now, a sense of euphoria, talkativeness, and courage to do things like dance or talk to someone you otherwise would not talk to if you were sober. That is described as having liquid courage in the previous chapter.

Uncharacteristic behavior, poor judgment, loss of balance, poor coordination, slurred speech, decreased visual acuity and blurred vision, nausea, vomiting, memory impairment, and being loud and obnoxious are common behaviors seen as blood alcohol concentrations continue to rise. Actions associated with continued drinking and increasing blood alcohol levels include confusion, disorientation, spinning sensation, inability to walk, incontinence of urine and feces, extreme sleepiness, decreased ability to breathe spontaneously, coma, respiratory arrest, and ultimately death.

I took the time to go through those behaviors again because it is imperative for you to have a good appreciation of the different signs of increasing levels of intoxication. Remember, as a person continues to drink, their level of intoxication becomes increasingly higher. They are not merely drunk, and it is important for you to understand that concept. Having an appreciation for the different levels of intoxication should help you to recognize how impaired someone may be, and empower you to make the right choices when dealing with that person who may be vulnerable and unable to care for himself or herself or make wise decisions.

Hopefully, if you drink, you will recognize you are becoming impaired and decide to stop drinking before you become too intoxicated to care for yourself. If you drink with friends, it may be a good idea to give them permission to keep you from drinking if they see you becoming increasingly impaired. This sort of goes along the same lines as having a designated driver and reinforces the fact that your intent is to drink responsibly and not drink to the point of becoming vulnerable and helpless.

Notice one of the behaviors mentioned above was memory impairment. Some of you may not believe this, but people have reported not remembering things after having just one or two drinks. Memory formation is a complex process that involves a variety of chemical interactions in different parts of the brain. A discussion of those complex interactions is beyond the scope of this book, but that information is available in textbooks and many articles you can find on the internet.

My intent is not to prepare you to become a neurologist, brain surgeon, or neuroscientist, but we do need to review the basics of memory formation so you can have an appreciation of why certain people don't remember things after a night of drinking. There's one area in the brain that you must remember when it comes to memory formation.

That area is called the hippocampus. The hippocampus is involved in memory formation, and alcohol interferes with that process. Without getting too technical and scientific, the main thing you should understand is that the hippocampus plays important roles in converting short-term memory into long-term memory. Alcohol's effect on memory is dose-dependent; meaning drinking larger quantities of alcohol may increase the chances of having the associated memory impairment.

One explanation of memory formation involves converting a sensory input, like talking to someone or experiencing some event like making out or having sex, and then transferring that sensory input into short-term memory. Once the short-term memory is formed, that memory is transferred into long-term memory. Long-term memories are stored and are retrievable for use in the future. To clarify this process, let's assume the brain works similar to a computer.

So you have to type a paper, and it takes you several days to complete the paper. You name the document and save it to your desktop or documents so you are able to find it when you want to continue writing. You complete the paper, and now have to turn it in. Where do you find it? Hopefully, you saved it correctly so you can retrieve it and turn it in.

You typing the information can be compared to the sensory input described above. Your computer should temporarily store what you are typing as you are typing it. This is similar to the brain converting sensory inputs into short-term memory. But what happens if you forget to hit the save button to actually save it? Saving the information does not happen automatically. You actually have to intentionally save it. Depending on the type of computer you have, that process may be different. Selecting the save function is similar to the brain encoding and transferring information from short-term memory into long-term memory.

Have you ever been working on a project and then forgot to save it? So let's say you forget to save it and then turn your computer off. What happens the next day when you try to retrieve what you wrote the day before? I'll tell you what happens. It's not there! You cannot find it, but you know you wrote it. You probably procrastinated and waited until the last minute to get it done. I know some of you reading this right now are laughing because you know what I'm talking about.

So what do you do now? Tell your boss or instructor your dog ate it or the little green people from outer space stole it from you? How about this one, "See what happened was, I was sick and spent the night in the emergency room." Some of you may be able to get away with excuses like that, but I don't think I could have ever been successful with something like that because I probably would have busted out laughing. You know like LOL or LMAO. How does this relate to the effects of alcohol on the brain and memory? Alcohol primarily interferes with the encoding or transfer of information from short-term memory to long-term memory.

Just as you are unable to retrieve something you typed if you don't save it, some people are unable to retrieve memories about things they did while they were intoxicated. Why do people forget to save important things they type? There could be a million reasons for this. Some people never forget to save their work, others do, and if you ask them what happened, they may say they thought they saved it and they just can't understand what happened. Similarly, some people never experience memory impairment after drinking, but others describe having memory impairment every time they drink.

Some people report having memory impairment after only having one or two drinks, and others say they have been intoxicated to the point of vomiting, room spinning, slurred speech, and even falling asleep, but they retained total recall of events that occurred during the drinking. Certain genetic factors and other variables have been linked to the probability of someone experiencing memory impairment after drinking. Binge drinking, consuming a large amount of alcohol within a short period of time, and a previous history of suffering memory impairment after drinking, are predictors of future episodes of experiencing memory impairment related to drinking.

Alcohol-related memory impairment is commonly referred to as a blackout. A blackout is strictly related to memory and is entirely separate from falling asleep or passing out from the effects of alcohol. People often think 'blackouts' are synonymous with 'passing out,' but that is a common mistake that deserves clarification.

Blackouts are not related to or dependent upon a state of consciousness. In fact, people who experience blackouts are fully awake, alert and engaged with others. They just don't remember what they did. Passing out, on the other hand, is directly related to a state of consciousness, and basically means a person is asleep secondary to the effects of the alcohol. Blackouts are described as being either 'fragmentary' or 'en bloc.' The fundamental difference is people who experience fragmentary blackouts can remember certain things that happened during a night of drinking, but they have gaps in their memory.

They remember bits and pieces of the events and can often retrieve additional information with cues from people who witnessed their behavior when they were intoxicated. En bloc blackouts differ because people who experience en bloc blackouts have no memory of events that happened after a certain point. Fragmentary blackouts are far more common than en bloc blackouts. Reviewing the scenario at the beginning of this chapter, the details describe someone who experienced a fragmentary blackout. He was binge drinking, undressed, was dancing on a table, and drove his car home.

Obviously, he was awake when he was dancing on the table, and it would have been impossible for him to drive home safely if he were asleep. Think about it, how could someone make left turns, right turns, stop at traffic lights, open the garage, and park the car if they were asleep? He did all of those things but does not remember doing them. He remembers certain details and may eventually remember more if his friends tell him what he actually did. His experience is a classic example of a fragmentary blackout. Alarmingly, many people have reported doing things during a night of drinking that they do not remember the next morning.

Some of the more worrisome behaviors include having sex with strangers, having unprotected intercourse, getting into fights, vandalism, destruction of property, having sex with friends, performing sexual acts that they would never do while sober, and waking up naked with someone in their bed. Often times, these incidents are so scary some people never drink again. Can you imagine how it would feel to wake up naked next to a stranger? To make things worse, what if you were to notice a hickey on your neck or feel sore in your vaginal, penile, or anal region? At that point, most people would be able to put two and two together and realize that some form of sexual contact happened with the stranger.

Does it mean you were raped if you don't remember actively participating with the stranger? What if the person in your bed is a friend or acquaintance? Should they have known you would not remember things the next morning? There is no way to tell if a person isn't going to remember the events that occurred during a night of drinking. Remember, blackouts specifically refer to memory impairment and are not dependent on one's state of consciousness or level of alertness. Everyone who was clapping for the guy in the scenario as he undressed and danced on the table was probably entertained by his actions. He probably even got a few high fives.

Many couples who engage in consensual intercourse after a night of drinking, report that one of them has memory impairment the following morning. Because they know each other and are in a relationship, they trust each other and may not feel violated if they don't remember having sex. There have been instances where an individual tells their friends that they have every intention of having sex with a particular person on a given night. The two meet at a club, have a few drinks, dance, make out on the dance floor, and decide to have sex. They spend the night together and have sex where both people seem to be consenting participants. They wake up the next morning, both naked and lying in each other's arms, and the person who previously told their friends they wanted to have sex with the other person has no memory of the events that took place after a certain point in the club. In fact, they may not even remember leaving the club. They especially don't remember consenting to or even having sex. Does that mean they were raped or sexually assaulted?

Many people would not classify that scenario as rape or sexual assault. Others, would. Regardless, many have been on trial and accused of sexual assault because someone said they did not remember consenting, and therefore, they must have been raped. At that point, the ultimate decision and fate of the accused is now in the hands of the jury. What will the jury think and how will they decide?

En bloc blackouts are less common, but they do occur. Using the same scenario, a classic example of an en bloc blackout would be if he remembered going to the party and having a drink, but then not remembering anything else afterward. After waking up the next morning, he would have no recollection of any of the events that happened at the party, and would not be able to retrieve any information, even with cues from his friends. Both fragmentary and en bloc blackouts result from alcohol's inhibiting effects on the hippocampus.

Interference with encoding and transferring of information from short-term to long-term memory is the primary problem. Fragmentary blackouts arise from an interruption and incomplete blockage of that process. En bloc blackouts result from a more permanent and total blockage. Information that is not encoded properly cannot be retrieved properly.

I think all will agree the best defense is awareness, education, and prevention. Awareness and education empower individuals to make smarter choices, and ultimately, prevent themselves from making poor decisions that lead to criminal prosecution and potential conviction.

7

WHY DO SOME PEOPLE FALL ASLEEP OR PASS OUT AFTER DRINKING AND IS IT OKAY TO HAVE SEX WITH SOMEONE WHO IS SLEEPING?

SCENARIO # 4

Several girls decide to get drunk. They purchase several six packs of beer and three bottles of liquor. They begin taking shots and chasing it with beer. One of the girls wants to show she can drink more than the others can, and so she continues to take shots repeatedly chasing each shot with beer.

Shortly afterward, she falls asleep on the floor and her friends have difficulty waking her up. They become alarmed because she is unresponsive. They call 911, and she is rushed to the local hospital emergency room.

Alcohol poisoning is a very serious condition that can lead to death if not recognized and treated properly. Many people don't realize alcohol can become a poison and a person can die if they drink enough of it.

There is a core difference between falling asleep after drinking and becoming unresponsive and unconscious after drinking. Because alcohol is a central nervous system depressant, people often begin to feel tired and sleepy after they reach a certain level of intoxication. Usually, although individuals who begin to feel sleepy or tired are intoxicated, they also are aware of what's going on.

They know they are intoxicated, and they know they are feeling tired. They know the best thing for them at the time is to lie down and go to sleep. They probably are still able to engage in conversations with their friends who may be asking them if they want to continue partying. They most likely realize they have had too much to drink and decline offers to keep partying. Just as they are able to refuse offers to continue partying, they are also probably able to reject offers for consensual sex.

At this stage of intoxication, it would not be unusual for an individual to have the ability to appreciate their surroundings, understand what others are saying to them, and have the capacity to accept or decline offers to do things. Even though they maintain that ability, they most likely would rather climb into bed and go to sleep. If someone attempted to sexually assault them at that moment, they would probably recognize what was happening, and would be able to voice that they are not interested in sex and just want to be left alone. Also, it would probably not be that difficult to wake them up from sleeping if it was necessary.

There becomes a point, however, when an individual is so intoxicated, they are unable to remain conscious. Their brain is so affected by the amount of alcohol they have consumed, they become unresponsive and unconscious. Not only will they be unresponsive, but also their breathing may be less than eight to ten breaths per minute, their heart rate can be severely slowed, their body temperature can drop significantly, and their gag reflex, which is involved in inducing vomiting to prevent aspiration and choking, becomes impaired.

Those symptoms are often recognized as alcohol poisoning, and also include other symptoms like confusion, cold and clammy skin, and vomiting while asleep. Unlike the individual who is merely sleeping because they are tired and sleepy after drinking, people who are unresponsive or unconscious are not able to appreciate their surroundings or participate in conversations. They are not able to decline offers or protect themselves from assault.

Having sex with someone in that condition is definitely a crime, and is commonly referred to as an aggravated sexual assault. What should you do if you suspect a friend of yours may be suffering from alcohol poisoning? Well, the first thing I recommend is to call 911 for help. Sometimes, this is not an easy call to make. Peer pressure may prevent someone from calling 911. Friends may not recognize the situation is serious and life threatening. They may think to call 911 is overkill and that calling 911 will bring unnecessary attention to the situation.

This becomes a bigger issue if the people drinking are underage. A typical scenario I have encountered is when a group of teenagers gather at someone's house because their parents are out of town. Somehow, alcohol shows up and everybody is drinking. Because they are trying to get a buzz, they binge drink, which means five or more drinks per two hours for males and four or more drinks per two hours for females, and they quickly become intoxicated.

Usually, someone wants to show how much he or she can drink, so they drink more than the others do. The next thing you know, that person is throwing up and eventually, passes out on the couch or the floor.

The rest of the group is now concerned because one of them is passed out and unresponsive. What do they do now? Do they call someone? Call their parents? Throw cold water on them? Just stand there and freak out?

The chatter usually goes something like this: Someone wake him up, OMG! He is not moving! I don't think he is breathing! I never should have been here. Let's all stay calm! I'm calling 911! No, stupid, if you call 911, we will all be in trouble. My dad is going to kill me. I'll be grounded for life! I'm out of here!

You see how difficult this can be?

So let me ask you this question. Would you rather do nothing and have your friend die right in front of your eyes or would you rather call 911 and save their life? Either way, 911 will eventually get a call. I think it's best for 911 to get the call when your friend is still alive as opposed to responding to take your friend to the morgue. Will you get in trouble for underage drinking and possibly get grounded when your parents find out? Probably. But don't you think it will be much worse if now you are being questioned by the police and potentially accused of contributing to your friend's death? Which would you prefer—grounded at home or arrested and taken to jail for contributing to your friend's death?

So you make the right decision and call 911. Now, what do you do before they arrive? You want to stay with your friend and never leave them by themselves. Try to wake them up, and if you are unable to wake them up, at least turn them on their side in case they vomit. Remember, their gag reflex is probably not working correctly, so if they vomit, it may block their airway, and they may choke on the vomit.

If they recently stopped drinking, their blood alcohol level may still be rising, and they will become increasingly impaired with time. I used the scenario of underage drinkers to describe why it may be difficult to call 911, but don't be misled by that scenario.

Many people twenty-one-years-old and older find themselves in the same situation. The common mistake is that friends don't recognize how serious the condition is. They think the person will sleep it off while everyone else continues to party. That may be true for the individual who is just tired and sleeping, but probably not true for the person who is unresponsive and unconscious.

It is never ok to have sex with someone who is sleeping, regardless of whether they are drinking or not. Someone who is sleeping is unable to give consent. If you make any form of sexual contact with someone who is sleeping, you have done so without his or her consent, which means you have committed a crime.

Sexual contact means things like touching their breasts, touching their buttocks, touching their vaginal or penile area, and it does not matter if they are fully clothed or not. Abusive sexual contact is any form of touching a person as described in the previous sentence without their consent. It does not matter if they are intoxicated, sober, awake, or sleeping.

If they are sleeping, do not touch them or try to engage in any form of sexual activity. If you do, be prepared to lose everything you have worked for because the police will be knocking at your door.

Now, if inappropriately touching someone when he or she is awake or asleep is a crime, what do you think about having sex with someone who is passed out, unresponsive, and unconscious? Having sex with someone who is passed out, unresponsive, or unconscious is definitely a crime. It doesn't matter if it's your boyfriend, girlfriend, or spouse. It doesn't matter if you have been in a sexual relationship with the person previously.

I have been involved in several cases where a boyfriend or girlfriend reported their significant other sexually assaulted them while they were sleeping or intoxicated to the point where they were unable to consent.

I have also been involved in several cases where married individuals accused their spouse of sexual assault because the spouse attempted or actually did have sex with the other while they were asleep. If you are convicted of sexually assaulting someone who is sleeping, or unable to give consent because they are intoxicated to the point of being unable to give consent, expect to go to prison and expect to be registered as a sex offender for the rest of your life.

8

CAN I HAVE SEX WITH SOMEONE IF WE BOTH HAVE BEEN DRINKING OR IS IT A CRIME?

SCENARIO # 5

A friend and I decide to go out. We have a few drinks and are having a good time at the bar. We both realize we are too intoxicated to drive home so we call a taxi.

Since we will not drive, we have a few more drinks while waiting for the taxi to arrive. We were both slurring our speech a little and both were a little off balance.

When we got back to my apartment, we went into my room and started making out. We had intercourse and we both seemed to enjoy it.

I know some of you can relate to that scenario. This situation happens all the time. People usually don't really need a reason to hang out with friends and have a few drinks.

This happens almost daily, and especially on the weekends and special occasions. It could be someone's birthday, getting together to watch the championship game, or the championship fight, celebrating graduation, celebrating finishing final exams, partying to bring in the

New Year, and about a million other reasons. Generally, people just like having a good time, and alcohol is usually available if people want to drink.

Typical scenario: Two people are physically attracted to each other, they start talking, and one of them says, "Hey, can I buy you a drink?" The other says, "Sure." Now they have a drink together. Seems pretty reasonable and ordinary, right? Or they are someplace where alcohol is provided so there is no need to buy someone a drink. It could be a house party, party at the workplace, party on a college campus, fraternity, or sorority party, and the list goes on and on. Ok, at this point, it appears no crimes have happened.

Guess what? There are many people out there who believe, after a person has one drink, they are unable to consent to sex. I'm even talking about after having one glass of wine with dinner. Many people don't drink, and so they are relying on what they have heard from other people or what they have read. We will come back to those people who don't drink, and I'll show you how someone who does not drink may have a significant impact on your life. Most people are completely aware of what they are doing and are able to consent to anything after having one drink.

If someone is drinking for the first time, he or she may become intoxicated to the point where they cannot consent to sex after having one or two drinks, but usually, it will be obvious to others that they are intoxicated to that point. So let's move forward in the evening. Now a few hours have passed and the two people have had a few drinks. They are now becoming really friendly toward each other and are having an excellent time. They may be gazing into each other's eyes and realizing the other person seems more attractive now than earlier in the night.

They may be laughing at each other's corny jokes, and talking about all the cool things they have done and plan to do. Having the ability to recognize they are too intoxicated to drive and deciding to call a taxi shows, even though they were intoxicated, they still had the critical judgment to call a taxi. At that point, they probably should have stopped drinking and just waited for the taxi to arrive.

Alcohol has a way of making people make unwise decisions, and some people would have made the unwise decision to drive themselves home. In that case, they would be driving under the influence of alcohol and would be breaking the law. So they wait for the taxi, have a few more drinks, and now began to slur their speech and become a little off balance. Does someone who is slurring his or her speech and walking off balance have the ability to consent to sex? Now the situation becomes more complicated.

What do you think the people who believe an individual cannot consent to sex after having one drink will think about someone who is slurring their speech and is off balance? Some of those who believe a person can consent to sex after having one drink may not be so sure now. They may feel that if a person is slurring their speech and off balance, they probably are too intoxicated to consent to sex. Do you care about those people who now, at this point, think consensual sex is out of the question? Hopefully, you will not find yourself in the position where their opinion matters to you.

So the couple now makes it back to the apartment, makes out, and has sex. Was it consensual sex or was it a crime? Now it really may be confusing to some of you. What is the correct answer? What do the people who actually had the sex think? Do both of them feel it was consensual? Does one of them regret having sex and now feel they have been taken advantage of? Will anyone believe it if one of the individuals was a male and the other a female and the male reports that he was unable to give consent and the female took advantage of him?

What if we are talking about same-sex couples? Can a woman be charged with rape if she has sex with another female who was too intoxicated to consent? Can a male be accused of rape if he has sex with another male who was too drunk to consent? Just recently, laws have been passed to protect victims in same sex relationships. So, yes, the correct answer to the question about same-sex couples and consent is the same as that for heterosexual couples. There have been cases of females being prosecuted for raping males, but that does not happen as often as males being prosecuted for raping females.

The most current language in some of the laws related to alcohol, sex, and consent use words and phrases like it's a crime if the person was unable to consent due to the effects of an intoxicant, if the person was incapacitated and if the person was unconscious. Ok, it's pretty obvious if the person is unconscious, but what does 'due to the effects of an intoxicant and incapacitated' mean? Inability to consent due to the impact of an intoxicant only means the person was intoxicated to the point of not being able to consent.

There is no magic button or another way to know for sure when a person who has been drinking crosses the point of being able to consent and not able to consent. I have evaluated and treated many individuals who say they were intoxicated to the point of slurring their speech, losing their balance, and vomiting, but they were still able to appreciate what was going on around them and able to consent to sex if they wanted. Intoxicated individuals sometimes make poor choices and do things they would never do when they are sober. Alcohol affects many parts of the brain, and one of those parts deals with critical judgment and making decisions.

Trying to decide if someone is too intoxicated to consent to sex should be a warning sign. If you have the slightest doubt about a person's ability to consent, do not initiate any sexual contact like touching or kissing, and definitely do not have sex with that person. I know some of you didn't like reading that and might have even been in a similar situation where you did have sex with a person you knew was intoxicated. That situation may have worked out fine for you, and it may have even been some of the best sex the both of you have ever had.

You may have wondered if they were too intoxicated to consent, but then convinced yourself although they were visibly intoxicated, they still had the ability to consent. Many others have made that same decision, and now are spending years sitting behind prison bars. Is it really worth it? I guess it depends on how you look at it. Some people may think they will never have the chance to have sex with that person again, so they are willing to take the risk. I strongly recommend against taking such a risk. Help the individual get home safe and let them know you care for them.

Even if they do have the ability to consent, they will

likely respect you for realizing they are intoxicated and taking care of them. You may even get lucky the next time when both of you are sober.

Incapacitated sometimes is described as when a person is unable to appreciate that sex is being considered, unable to communicate their unwillingness to participate, and unable to physically protect themselves to avoid the sex.

Some people say if the other person didn't say no, then it's ok to have sex. Others think there should be a requirement for both people to say yes prior to sex. We have all heard 'No Means No' and understand if a person says no, the activity should stop, and if it doesn't, then the activity is considered forcible rape. Forcible rape involves some degree of actual physical force like violence and overpowering. It can also include forms of intimidation, the threat of bodily harm, or causing a degree of fear that makes the victim unable to defend themselves.

What about those who think both people should have to say yes? Let's explore what 'Yes means Yes' really means. Basically, it means that both people have to verbally communicate they want to engage in sex by saying the word yes. Some people have even gone as far as standing next to each other and sending each other a text message showing that they both consent to having sex.

I'm not sure what that does for being spontaneous, but at least it is documented in a text message that consent was mutual. People laugh at me all the time when I talk about sending text messages so there is proof both individuals agreed to consensual sex. They say it is not realistic, and that most people are not going to stop in the heat of the moment to send a text. I've talked to females who said it would be a turn off if a guy sent them a text message. They felt it would ruin the mood and make them not want to have sex. Several males and females said they would not mind it at all if someone suggested sending a text message. They felt, with all the people being accused of rape and sexual assault, a text message showing they both consented to the sex would be appropriate and would not be a turn-off.

Ok, let's consider this scenario: Two people are making out and on their way to having sex. One of them stops and says, "Hey, let me send you a text message asking you if you want to have sex and then you respond saying that you do so we both can be protected just in case one of us later thinks it was nonconsensual." I guess that would be great evidence in court to show the sex was consensual, but would the sex actually happen if someone did that? Would you consider it a turn-off? I actually think asking the other person if you can kiss them, make out with them and have sex with them is a good idea. It shows you respect their desires and you are asking for their permission, rather than assuming they want to be kissed, touched, or have sex with you.

By asking them the question, you give them the opportunity to say yes or no. If they say yes, you have their permission to proceed, and if they say no, you can now go take a cold shower and call it a night.

So now, let's get back to those people who think someone cannot consent to sex after having one drink and those who think if a person slurs their speech, loses their balance, or vomits, they cannot consent to sex. If you are accused of having sex with someone who says they were unable to consent due to the effects of an intoxicant, you will probably end up in court. During your trial, the jury will be selected.

What do you think the person who says someone can't consent to sex after having one drink will think when he or she hears the person accusing you had several drinks and was slurring their speech? What about jury members who think a person cannot consent to sex if they are intoxicated to the point of losing their balance and vomiting? Why put yourself in that situation? I know some of you may be desperate and may not ever get another chance to have sex in your life. (That was a joke, and I hope you are laughing.)

Seriously though, take my advice, and do not try to interpret whether or not someone has the ability to consent. If you have to think about it, they may have the capacity to consent, but trust me—it's not worth the risk.

9

WHAT OPTIONS DO I HAVE IF, AFTER A NIGHT OF DRINKING, I KNOW I HAVE BEEN RAPED?

Deciding what to do if you know you have been raped can be a difficult process. Some of you may not understand what I am saying, and you may think the decision should be very clear. I have spoken to many individuals who are confused about what they should do, and that confusion can be related to several factors.

Some people may think it is their fault because they were drinking, and so they may try to justify the rape. It is never the rape victim's fault. If you have been raped, the circumstances surrounding the rape do not justify you being raped. Others may have difficulty because they fear the negative attention they might be exposed to if they report the incident. Some fear no one will believe them because there were no witnesses, and it will basically come down to their word against the word of the accused.

I listed three common reasons that lead to confusion for some people, but there are many other reasons that could make that decision a difficult one. Regardless of the reason, I really want you to understand some people know they have been raped and they are unsure of what to do about it. When I say they know they have been raped, I'm not talking about those who were intoxicated to the point where they have significant memory impairment and really do not know what actually happened.

Additionally, I'm not talking about those situations where an individual is unsure of whether the sex was consensual or not. I'm specifically referring to situations where, even though drinking was involved, it is clear that an individual was taken advantage of and raped.

In that situation, two individuals are involved—the rape victim and the rapist. If you know you have been raped, I strongly recommend you call 911 or call the police to report the rape. By calling the police, you will get immediate assistance from the authorities who will also most likely be involved in investigating your case. Additionally, they will probably take you to the hospital so you can get immediate medical attention. Again, many people choose not to seek medical attention and many choose not to report the rape. Even if you decide not to report the rape, I strongly recommend you seek immediate medical attention.

Understand that the medical evaluation will be more detailed if the medical staff knows you are a rape victim. If they know you are a rape victim, the evaluation will not only be targeted toward treating you as a patient, but will also include other procedures to collect evidence to help the police identify the person who raped you. There are several reasons why seeking immediate medical attention is so important. You will be evaluated and tested for potential medical complications so you can receive the appropriate treatment. It is very important that you *not* take a shower or bath and *not* change your clothes or underwear prior to calling the police.

When you get to the medical facility, the evaluation will include gathering your clothes to check for any evidence that can be used to help investigate the case. You will also be evaluated for sexually transmitted diseases, pregnancy for females, tears, swelling, and bleeding in the vaginal, penile, or anal area, and other physical and psychological problems related to the rape.

You will likely be asked to give a blood sample, urine sample, and maybe even a saliva sample. One of the tests that may be performed on your blood sample is your blood alcohol concentration. Your blood alcohol concentration can be a very important test. By determining your blood alcohol concentration as close in time to the rape, doctors can evaluate your level of intoxication and give medical opinions on what behaviors you were possibly able to perform based on your level of intoxication at the time of the rape.

The evaluation most likely will also include taking pictures of any bruises or other identifying marks, using a cotton swab to collect a DNA sample from your mouth, vagina for females, penis for males, and anal areas. I have been involved in many cases where the rapist was convicted because of all the evidence that was collected shortly after the rape. I also have been involved in many cases where the rapist was convicted after being accused of rape months and years after the rape. Delayed reporting is essentially when the victim does not report the rape until some time after the rape actually occurred.

In those cases of delayed reporting, some of the victims did actually receive medical treatment, and some did not. I believe cases that involve delayed reporting may be harder to prove. For instance, if there was no evidence collected, no medical exam, and months or years have passed since the rape occurred, the police may feel they don't have enough evidence to prosecute the case.

Contrarily, I have seen cases that involved delayed reporting, where it was basically the alleged victim's word against the accused's word, and some of those cases resulted in a conviction. Based on my experience, and the cases I have been involved with, I recommend reporting the rape to the police as soon as it happens, and I also recommend getting a complete medical evaluation as soon as possible after the rape.

Delayed reporting is better than not reporting at all and can still result in the rapist being convicted and going to prison. Just realize delayed reporting seems counterintuitive to some people, and they may not understand why someone would delay in reporting they were raped. Because of that lack of understanding, the delayed report may not be taken as seriously by some, and the allegations may or may not be harder to prove depending on all of the factors associated with the case. Hopefully, you will never find yourself in a position where you have been raped, but if you do, just remember you do have options.

Some in that position choose to do nothing and attempt to justify it or find ways to deal with it. Some choose to discuss it with their close friends or family members. Others report it to the police immediately, and some report it to the police after some period of time has passed. I have given my recommendation above, and I stand by that advice to report it immediately and to get a full medical examination.

If you find yourself in that situation, you will have to make a decision. I'm sure your decision will be based on several factors and you will do what you feel is best for you. Even though I think it is best to report it immediately, I have evaluated and treated many patients who said they had been raped previously and chose not to report it. Although I disagree with that choice, it was their decision, and I respect them for making the decision they felt was in their best interest.

Sometimes, getting advice from family members, friends, and medical providers can help make the decision clearer and less confusing.

The last thing I'll say on this topic is to remember there is help out there for you if you are a victim of rape. You may experience anxiety, depression, posttraumatic stress disorder, and in some cases, even suicidal thoughts. Please don't go through this by yourself. Reach out to your family and friends, and talk to a mental health professional if you are experiencing sadness, anxiety, or problems with intimacy and interpersonal relationships.

10

WHAT SHOULD I DO IF I AM BEING ACCUSED OF HAVING INTERCOURSE WITH SOMEONE WHO SAYS THEY WERE TOO DRUNK TO CONSENT?

SCENARIO # 6

A few months after a night of drinking and having intercourse with a friend, I am contacted by the authorities and told that my friend reported I had raped her. What should I do?

Some of you may be thinking it's impossible to be accused of sexually assaulting someone months after you thought you had consensual sex with that individual. Well, let me set the record straight and keep it real for you. I have been involved in cases where people have been accused years after they had sex with an individual. Yes, that is correct—years afterward. I have been involved in cases where it basically boils down to her word versus his word, but the case still ended up in court, and the jury made a decision based on what they felt the evidence proved beyond a reasonable doubt.

If someone makes an allegation against you, saying you raped them or had sex with them without their consent, several things are going to happen before you are even contacted by the police. The police will interview the person who is making the allegation against you and try to gather any evidence that can be used to help them get a clearer picture of what actually transpired between the two of you. They may talk to people who know you and may ask your accuser to identify any people who may have information related to the allegations.

At some point, they will contact you and ask you to come into the police station for an interview. Based on the nature and the timing of the allegation, you may actually be arrested and processed at the local police station. That processing may include taking your photograph, formally known as taking your mug shot, taking your fingerprints, and gathering other personal information about you. They may even collect your DNA by swabbing inside your mouth with a cotton swab.

If they arrest you, they will read you your rights and tell you that anything you say can be used against you in a court of law. So what rights do you have? Well, the most important right you have is the right to speak to an attorney and to have an attorney present when the police ask you questions. You definitely want to cooperate with the police and not be hostile or belligerent, but at the same time, you should seriously consider working with them *after* speaking to an attorney.

This will probably be your first time ever being accused of a crime and your first time dealing with law enforcement. There may be many things you don't completely understand about the process, and things you have no idea you should even ask. You may think you fully understand because you have watched every episode of all the television shows dealing with the police, but in actuality, there may be things you are unfamiliar with.

Because of those reasons, it may be to your benefit to have a good working knowledge of the process prior to moving forward with your complete cooperation with the police. By obtaining an attorney, you give yourself the opportunity to talk with someone who is very familiar with the process and can educate you on the process. Don't feel like you are not cooperating with the police if you exercise your right to speak to an attorney.

I have worked with some people who said they felt forced into talking to the police prior to having an attorney, and they said they really didn't understand all the legal terminology and things the police were asking them. They felt they were at a disadvantage because they wanted to cooperate but didn't realize what they were dealing with. Some of them said they were told they could leave after talking with the police, but if they wanted to wait for an attorney, they would be there for an extended amount of time.

Some of the people I have worked with said they didn't think they could afford an attorney so they thought having an attorney was not an option. Everyone has the right to an attorney, and if you cannot afford one, one will be appointed for you. In most places, there are attorneys called public defenders who represent people who do not have the money to hire an attorney. It may seem like everyone on television has their own attorney, but in reality, many people do not have an attorney because they never had the need for a lawyer.

If you have the money to hire an attorney, you can be more selective in who you choose to represent you. If you do not have the money to hire an attorney, one will be provided for you. Based on all the cases I have been involved with over the years, and all the people I have spoken to about this topic, my recommendation is to inform the police you want to speak to an attorney prior to answering any questions the police may have for you.

I make that recommendation because of the number of people who said they felt unprepared to speak to the police and that they felt they were under-informed about the process. As I said earlier, I recommend fully cooperating with the police, and the police may be able to answer any questions you may have about the process. However, I still recommend having an attorney who can educate you on the process and speak on your behalf. I don't see any harm that can come to you by having an attorney from the outset.

Contrarily, you could potentially be harmed if you don't fully understand what you are being asked by the police and you misunderstand what they are asking you. You may think you are answering a certain question, but because you don't fully understand what is being asked, your response to the question may not be accurate.

Why take the chance of engaging in a conversation with the police when you are confused and not exactly sure what you are being asked? Let them know you want to fully cooperate, but you also respectfully wish to consult with an attorney first to ensure you are well informed of your rights and able to ask the attorney any questions you may have. Many people have declined their right to a lawyer and found themselves being interrogated by the police for multiple hours.

Speaking to an attorney and having an attorney present when you talk to the police may delay things, but it is the smart thing to do. Being accused of sexual assault is very serious, and if convicted, you will go to prison. If you did nothing wrong and are being falsely accused, get the advice of an attorney who has your best interest at heart.

So let me be very clear. Exercise your right to an attorney prior to answering questions from the police and giving a statement. If you still don't understand, you will see that advice again in the next section.

11

ADVICE FROM THE AUTHOR

This book was written to increase awareness about the devastating effects of alcohol, specifically related to the ability to consent to sex. My primary goal is prevention. Increased awareness leading to prevention is essential. So many lives are ruined secondary to behaviors associated with the debilitating effects of alcohol. I am confident we must increase our efforts to empower the masses through awareness and education. As a Forensic Psychiatrist and Family Medicine Physician, I have evaluated and treated many people with alcohol-related disorders.

Many have lost their careers, families, and their lives by not drinking responsibly. Through increased awareness, education, and treatment, many have recovered from their losses and now lead productive lives. People of all ages can become victims of the consequences of drinking irresponsibly. I have personally witnessed people die from alcohol-related liver disease, have evaluated and treated people with alcohol-related sexual trauma, and have seen well-intended people go to prison for many years because they lacked awareness about the intoxicating effects of alcohol and made poor choices.

This book was intended for both people who drink alcohol and their families and friends. We all have to do a better job of increasing alcohol awareness in hopes that we can influence behavior and prevent someone from making the mistakes so many make every day. For the person who drinks and becomes intoxicated to the point of not being able to remain in control of the situation, I challenge you to change your drinking habits before it's too late.

Too many people are reported missing or have been found brutally raped and beaten, and they have no memory of what actually happened because they were intoxicated to the point of either experiencing a blackout or even passing out. If they survive the trauma, their lives are severely changed, and they have to fight every day to improve their quality of life. If you are going to drink, drink responsibly and avoid binge drinking. To the person who is underage, less than twenty-one-years-old, it is illegal for you to drink and my advice is that you do not drink.

However, I know many people begin drinking when they are teenagers, and many teenagers who read this book will probably continue to drink. Some high school students have told me that alcohol is readily available to them and that more than fifty to sixty percent of high school students actually have experimented with alcohol. Many lose their lives driving under the influence of alcohol, and many are involved in alcohol-related sexual assaults.

My hope is that by providing increased awareness of how alcohol affects the brain and exposing teenagers to more of the negative consequences related to underage drinking, some will decide not to drink and influence their peers to also not drink. To the people who have experienced an alcohol blackout, realize you will likely continue to have blackouts if you continue your same drinking habits.

Binge drinking increases your chances of having a blackout, and many people have done things they regret but have no memory of doing those things. Some people never drink again after experiencing a blackout and being told what they actually did while intoxicated. Drinking responsibly will decrease the likelihood of you continuing to have blackouts, and I sincerely hope you change your drinking habits before you find yourself in a compromising situation like being raped, assaulted, or having unintended and unsafe sex with a stranger.

To the person who is considering having sex with someone who is intoxicated, please reconsider and wait until you both are sober. You both may be intoxicated and able to consent, but it is not worth the risk of being accused of having sex with someone who was unable to consent.

If you think you have been raped, please report it to the authorities and seek medical treatment. I know many do not report, and I'm sure they have their reasons. Never have sex with someone who is sleeping or unconscious. It is a crime.

If you are accused of having sex with someone who is unable to consent, cooperate with the police, but only after exercising your right to an attorney.

For the family and friends of people who drink, you will be affected if your loved one or friend becomes a victim of an alcohol-related incident. Talk with them about the information in this book so they can become more aware. They will probably come to you if they get themselves into trouble or have questions. Familiarize yourself with the information in this book so you can discuss it with them when they ask for your help.

I am often called into court as an expert witness to explain the effects of alcohol on the brain to the jury. I also have served as a consultant for the prosecution and the defense. In all the cases I have been involved in, one thing remains the same—the alleged victims of alcohol-related rape and sexual assault and their families have a difficult time during the trial.

Sometimes, the trial happens months or even years after the alleged rape. The pain and suffering they experience is still very evident. Likewise, the accused and their family have experienced a similar pain and suffering. The jury will decide the verdict, but the verdict cannot erase all the pain and suffering experienced by the alleged victim, the accused, and their families and friends. That is why we must increase our efforts on prevention.

We can make a difference if we work together. Collectively, we can join forces to increase awareness and education. Let's proactively get the word out rather than reactively responding to the bad news.

It has truly been a pleasure writing this book, and I sincerely hope you were enlightened by the content. If you are more aware of the devastating effects of alcohol on the brain, more aware of the different levels of intoxication, feel empowered to avoid becoming a victim of an alcohol-related sexual assault, or feel empowered to drink responsibly and treat others with dignity and respect by asking for permission before engaging in any form of sexual activity—then the objective of this book has been met.

There has been a lot of focus on sexual assaults in the media recently and rightfully so. Use the information in this book to help address the problem. Give it as a gift to your loved one as they transition from your home into the next chapter of their life. I'm sure they will thank you for it. Prevention is key!

DR. MARSHALL SMITH

Dr. Marshall Smith has been practicing medicine for eighteen years. After completing combined residency training in General Psychiatry and Family Medicine in Washington, D.C., he obtained board certification from both The American Board of Psychiatry and Neurology and The American Board of Family Medicine. He did clinical work for four years prior to returning to Washington, D.C. to complete a Forensic Psychiatry Fellowship. He is currently a board certified Forensic Psychiatrist.

During his fellowship training, Dr. Smith evaluated hundreds of patients at several esteemed locations including The Behavioral Analysis Unit of the FBI, Quantico, Virginia; Maryland's maximum security forensic psychiatric hospital; Clifton T. Perkins Hospital Center, Jessup, Maryland; and the Adult Forensic section of St. Elizabeth's Hospital, Washington, D.C.

Dr. Smith has consulted on and testified in court cases across North America, Europe, and Asia. He serves as an expert witness in a wide variety of cases and has extensive clinical experience working with patients with substance abuse problems. Dr. Smith has evaluated and treated many patients with alcohol-related disorders over the past fifteen years, and as an expert witness, he has educated multiple juries on how alcohol affects human behavior.

In his position as Clinical Consultant for two separate Substance Abuse Programs, Dr. Smith treated patients diagnosed with alcohol-related disorders individually and in group settings. His knowledge and experience as both a forensic psychiatrist and family physician make him highly sought after by prosecutors and defense attorneys across the United States.

You can contact Dr. Smith via email:
alcoholexpert4u@yahoo.com

www.ingramcontent.com/pod-product-compliance
Lightning Source LLC
Chambersburg PA
CBHW030727180526
45157CB00008BA/3072